Simple Snatch Programming for Kettlebells:

Dominate the 100 Rep Snatch Test

By

Zakary Morris

PUBLISHED BY Wandering Girevik Publications LLC,
Copyright 2021

wanderinggirevik@gmail.com

ISBN: 9798498275857

Published in the United States of America

DISCLAIMER

The information contained in this publication is for educational purposes only and is not designed to and does not provide medical, nutritional, or health advice, diagnosis, or opinion for any health or individual problem. The material presented is not a substitute for medical or other professional health services from a qualified health care provider who is familiar with the unique facts of the individual, and should not be used in place of a visit, call, consultation, or advice of a physician or healthcare provider. Individuals should always consult with a qualified health care provider about any health concern and prior to undertaking any new treatment. The publisher assumes no responsibility and specifically disclaims all liability for any consequence relating directly or indirectly to any action or inaction that a reader takes based on any information contained herein.

Neither the publisher nor the authors are engaged in rendering professional advice or services to the individual reader. The ideas, procedures, and suggestions contained in this book are not intended as a substitute for consulting with a physician. All matters regarding health require medical supervision. Neither the authors nor the publisher shall be liable or responsible for any loss or damage allegedly arising from any information or suggestion in this book.

Be advised that no one should undertake exercises in the nature of those addressed in this book without prior consultation with a physician. Nor does the publisher make any representations concerning whether any of the exercises or suggestions provided by the trainers or physical fitness specialists featured in this book would be effective or appropriate for the reader's needs or expectations. The publisher expressly disclaims any and all responsibility and/or liabilities that might result from the uninformed or misinformed application of the techniques identified herein as well as for any unsupervised physical fitness training.

While the authors have made every effort to provide accurate contact information at the time of the publication, neither the publisher nor the authors assume any responsibility for errors, or for changes that occur after publication. Further, the publisher does not have any control over and does not assume any responsibility for the author or third-party websites or their content.

Finally, the publisher disclaims any and all liabilities arising from the use of any equipment featured in this book and makes no representations as to the safety, utility, or adequacy of the equipment generally or with respect to any specific purpose.

Introduction

The following manual is intended for individuals who are seeking to not only complete the 100 rep kettlebell snatch test in under a 5 minute timeframe, but also the ability to do so on a regular basis. It is my belief that if a human being is able to acquire the ability to complete this feat on any given day, even to the extent that little or no warm-up is needed, that he or she will possess the strength and stamina for anything physical that they will need accomplish in regard to everyday life. It will also be of tremendous use for those who aspire to earn an instructor certification from an organization that requires the successful completion of the snatch test.

There are many things that this manual is **not**, however. It is not a magic program that will guarantee results within a particular timeframe or an approach that can be utilized in order to meet a goal that involves a deadline that must be met between now and a specific date in the future. The concepts presented here are **perpetual** in nature and do not have any regard for meeting any sort of deadline. Instead, the focus is placed upon the lifelong pursuit of improving and perfecting the ability to perform the snatch effectively. The primary concern is simply improving snatch efficiency over a period of months if not years with the understanding that at some unspecified time in the future, the athlete will eventually reach a point in his or her life where the 100 rep snatch test can be completed habitually. I am a firm believer that organic results are much more rewarding and sustainable than forced results. When incremental improvements are made no matter how tiny they appear to be at the time of making them, each of these small steps will eventually add up to make an enormous difference as years go by. Winning the long game is what counts above all else. Always keep in mind that many sport specific training cycles which are focused on "peaking" are only for the purpose of coming in first place for a competition, **they are not always designed for longevity or injury prevention.** As Stan "Rhino" Efferding once said: "If you want to be healthy, don't compete."

If you have the ambition of competing in Girevoy Sport which involves peaking for a meet within a certain timeframe, I would highly recommend hiring a coach that can accommodate your immediate needs. If it is your intention to earn a kettlebell instructor certification that requires successful completion of the snatch test, then it is my conviction that the prospective candidate should possess the ability to complete the test in convincing fashion before registering for a course. Kettlebell certifications through a reputable organization are not to be underestimated, and hoping that you will pass all of the requirements without prior skill development is no different than cramming for a college exam the night before the test. When you do not make it a priority to study the course material as soon as the professor has assigned it to you, then more than likely you will fail the exam when the time comes. Waiting until the last minute is **never** a wise choice. Train until you can confidently pass the snatch test before you even entertain the idea of registering for a certification and don't put the cart before the horse.

With these expectations in mind, I firmly believe that the concepts and the principles that I will expand upon can be highly effective for improving the snatch so long as they are consistently adhered to and progress is thoroughly measured and recorded. There are many ways to achieve the ability to snatch a kettlebell for 100 repetitions in under 5 minutes, and the methods to follow are a very simple and straightforward way of reaching this goal.

Personal Accomplishments

In regard to my personal snatching accomplishments, at the time of writing this I have been able to complete the following:

- 102 rep snatch test (51 each arm) with a 24kg/53lb. kettlebell in 3:54 minutes, resting one minute and then completing 101 burpees in 8:58 minutes after doing so.
- 100 rep snatch test (50 each arm) with a 32kg/70.5 kettlebell in 4:05 minutes

- 121 rep snatch test (60 right, 61 left) with a 32kg/70.5 kettlebell in 5:43 minutes
- 68 reps (34 each arm) with a 40kg/88lb. kettlebell in 3:18 minutes
- 40 reps (20 each arm) with a 48kg/106lb. kettlebell in 1:50 minutes

All of these attempts consist of only one hand switch without putting the bell down. I have recorded footage of each of these attempts on my Instagram page (wandering_girevik) as well. In addition, I have also successfully completed the Simple & Sinister challenge which is a great feat of strength and endurance by its own merit. My height is 6' 3'' and my bodyweight can range from 203lbs. – 213lbs. depending on the time of year and the goals that I want to accomplish.

Pre-Requisites

This manual presumes that the athlete has already acquired basic proficiency as it pertains to kettlebell movements, such as:

- Deadlift (One and Two Handed)
- Swings (One and Two Handed)
- Cleans
- Presses
- The snatch itself.

It is not geared toward beginners, but rather novice-to-intermediate kettlebell lifters who have already mastered the ability to perform the exercise safely while possessing a desire to achieve and maintain a level of conditioning that is beyond that of the average human being. Many certifications require the ability to perform the full snatch for at least 5 clean repetitions on each side to perfection before having the ability to continue to the snatch test. The expectation is that the prospective athlete has time within his or her schedule to train for at least 2 to 3 times per week, including the ability to perform some of the assistance movements that will be recommended near the end of this manual. Another assumption is that you will have easy access to approximately 2-4 kettlebells as the programming requirements involve the use of at least two kettlebells which are approximately 12kg to 16kg apart in weight.

Why the Snatch?

Even as obtainable as I believe it to be, if the athlete has the ability to "knock out" the 100 rep snatch test as if it were second nature, they will be in better physical condition than at least 95% of people on the planet, possibly even more than that. There are very few movements that an athlete can perform which test muscular endurance, lung capacity, mental concentration, and will power more than the one arm snatch with the kettlebell. The better that you can become at snatching, then in turn you will also become better at everything else from the psychological benefits alone.

In comparison to other forms of cardiovascular conditioning, the snatch is exceptional in regard to its **measurability**. With long distance running, sprinting, sled dragging, or prowler pushing, the athlete is forced to find creative ways to run faster or increase distance, and this can often times be very challenging. With an exercise like the snatch however, we can whittle how progress is measured all the way down to a single repetition of the exercise. If an athlete wishes to improve his or her stamina, it is much easier to go from 20 to 21 repetitions while improving the snatch rather than to decrease a one mile run time by 10 seconds for example. Unless the athlete is a runner, then the kettlebell snatch can be a much more sensible alternative because its measurability involves much greater precision. In addition, it is far more convenient to snatch a kettlebell in a small corner of your home rather than jogging around a track or neighborhood, especially during colder months.

In an ideal world, every man and woman of able body would be able to complete the 100 rep snatch test within a 5 minute timeframe based upon their "test" weight as determined by a certifying organization. Even if your goal is simply to burn fat and look better, more than likely you will have very little body fat by normalizing this feat of conditioning as long as quality nutritional habits have been established.

Hardstyle Cast Iron vs. Competition Steel

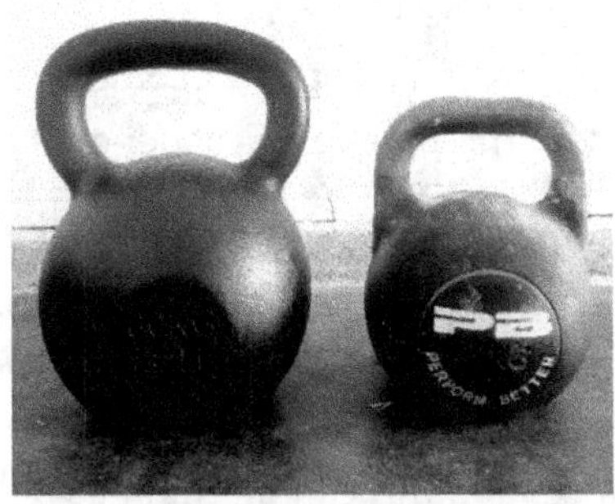

If you've trained with kettlebells long enough, you've more than likely become acquainted with the different designs of kettlebells that you can choose from. Although there is some variation here and there, they can generally be classified in one of two categories.

The first category is the cast iron or "hardstyle" kettlebell. This style of kettlebell is designed with a handle that is wide and the sides of the handle are rounded and extend outward. This handle design makes the hardstyle kettlebell superior for movements such as two handed swings, goblet squats, and one legged (pistol) squats. There is more room for both hands to perform two handed swings, and the hands can be placed underneath where the handle rounds out so that you will not lose your grip while perform goblet and pistol squats. As each kettlebell increases in weight, the circumference of the bell and the width of the handle also increases in size.

The second category is the stainless steel or "competition" kettlebell. These kettlebells are used in Girevoy (Russian Kettlebell) Sport and are designed with a slightly thinner, rectangular handle in which the sides of the handle are vertical rather than rounding outward. The open space between the dimensions of the handle, also known as the "window," is typically smaller in comparison to the hardstyle kettlebell. This handle design makes the competition kettlebell superior for cleaning, pressing, and snatching because it is much easier to insert the hand and wrist into the corner of the handle. As each kettlebell increases in weight, the circumference of the bell **does not** increase in size. It may increase very slightly up to a certain point, but it is kept as minimal as possible.

Overall, and particularly as it pertains to the snatch, I am quite candid in stating that I prefer **competition kettlebells**. Most distributors in the United States do not make a competition style bell past a 48kg in weight, otherwise they would be the only style that I would purchase. Although it would be advantageous to have some hardstyle bells for improving the pistol squat, the competition style bells can be used for, or are generally superior for, just about everything else. They are more expensive, but they are far less strenuous on joints, ligaments, and tendons along with being less likely to tear your hands. This is important because the less stress on the hands and joints, the greater the work capacity that can be produced and the more repetitions that can be performed. Another factor to consider is that stainless steel generally does not begin to rust as quickly as cast iron. Even if you intend on certifying through an organization that incorporates the hardstyle method, the dimensions of a competition kettlebell have excellent transferability to a 32kg sized cast iron which is the heaviest kettlebell that is used to test the snatch.

Simply put, you get what you pay for and it may be a wise choice to invest in competition bells as they are less injurious and will last a lifetime if properly taken care of.

Snatching Styles

Similar to how kettlebells typically come in two different designs, there are also two different styles of the snatch: The Hardstyle Method and the Girevoy Sport (GS) method. For the purpose of saving time, we won't go into too much detail concerning the nuances of each method as the manual presumes that the reader is already familiar with the movement. There are plenty of instructional videos that are widely available in order to teach them properly.

The Hardstyle snatch is predicated upon **maximum muscle recruitment.** It emphasizes the athlete's ability to use the mind in order to connect with as many supporting muscles as possible throughout the entire kinetic chain in an effort to move the kettlebell as explosively as possible. The heels of the feet are planted throughout each repetition, the shoulders remain even and packed, and the working arm moves out and up as vertically as possible. When the concentric (upward) portion of the snatch has been completed and the back is, the kettlebell is "thrown forward" similar to shooting a basketball while ensuring that the handle is caught by the mid-knuckles while moving past the callus line on the hand on the way down. This style of snatching places a great deal of emphasis the glutes, quads, and hips.

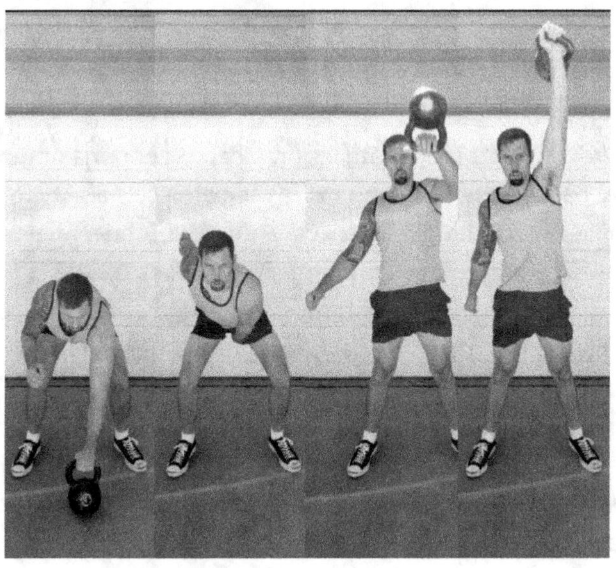

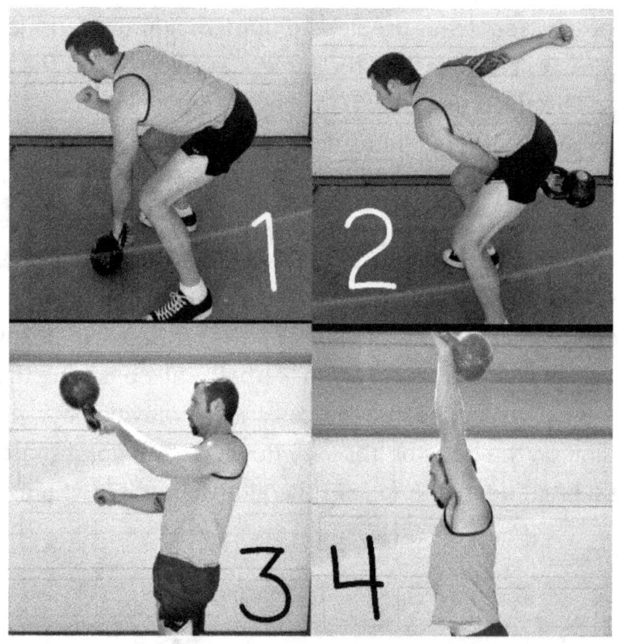

The Girevoy Sport (GS) snatch is predicated upon **maximum energy conservation.** It emphasizes the athlete's ability to use the mind in order to pinpoint every nuance of the movement pattern so that the most amount of repetitions can be performed within a specific timeframe regardless of explosiveness or muscular development. Rather than maintaining a very rigid stance throughout each repetition, the GS athlete will often make "rocking" movements while performing the snatch. The heel that is on the same side of the working arm will elevate during the concentric (upward) portion of the movement while both heels may elevated on the eccentric (downward) portion of the movement, although this can vary depending on the athlete's preference. This creates a sort of "1, 2, 3" rhythm and pacing during the snatch. The handle of the kettlebell is "pulled" upward while it is presented at either a 45 degree angle or vertically rather than horizontally, and the space between the thumb and index finger is inserted into the corner of the handle while simultaneously locking out the elbow and fixating into the overhead position. On the way down, the hand and wrist turn the kettlebell outward and transition the handle from the palm to the mid-knuckles rather than throwing it completely forward as demonstrated in the hardstyle snatch.

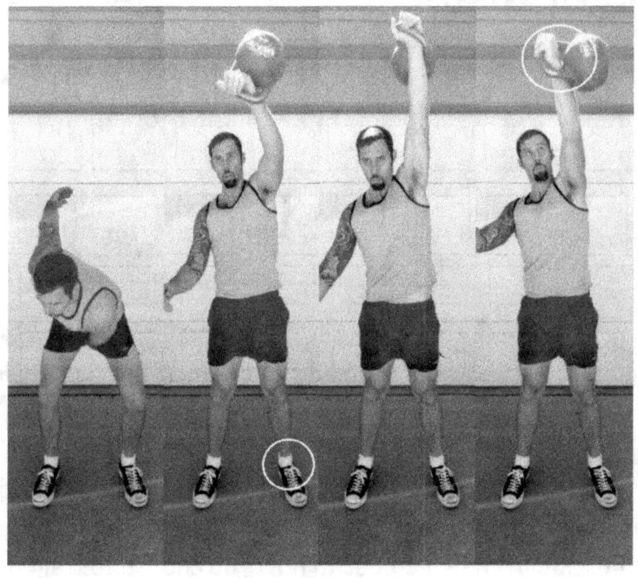

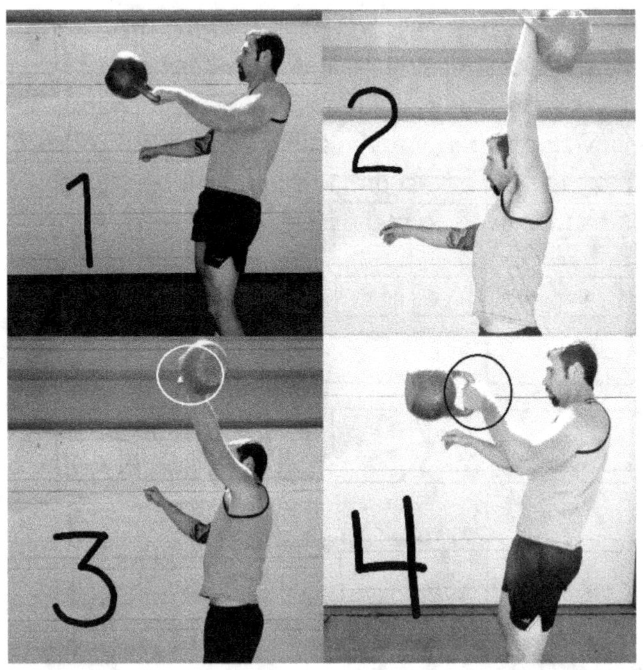

In regard to each style of snatching, neither is superior to the other and are dependent upon the athlete and the unique goals that he or she has in mind. Rather than thinking dichotomously, it can also be of great benefit to **incorporate elements of both styles.** There is more than one way to skin a catfish, and dogma need not apply when it comes to how you choose to train or experiment unless you are required to follow strict guidelines as prescribed by a coach. Personally, I have used a hybrid of both styles over the years, leaning toward a predominantly hardstyle snatch with some GS techniques added which has worked with great success.

Helpful Techniques and Nuances to Consider

In regard to experimenting with the snatch, there are some nuances that you may want to entertain the idea of incorporating while working toward the 100 rep snatch test, especially as you begin to progress in weight. I would also add that it is very useful to **record your lifting.** You would be amazed at what sort of technical improvements that you could uncover by reviewing recorded attempts and making corrections afterward.

As previously mentioned, my style of snatching is predominantly hardstyle with some GS techniques added. This consists of two distinct characteristics in particular:

- Rather than swinging the arm completely outward on the way up and throwing the kettlebell forward on the way down, pull the handle upward while it is facing you at a 45 degree angle and insert the space between the thumb and index finger into the corner of the handle. Turn the kettlebell outward and transition the handle from the palm to the mid-knuckles rather than throwing it completely forward. In other words, **"GS" the upper body and "Hardstyle" the lower body.** Adding this nuance to the hardstyle snatch will go a long way when it comes to saving your wrists and not tearing your hands, providing the ability to perform more repetitions and train more often.

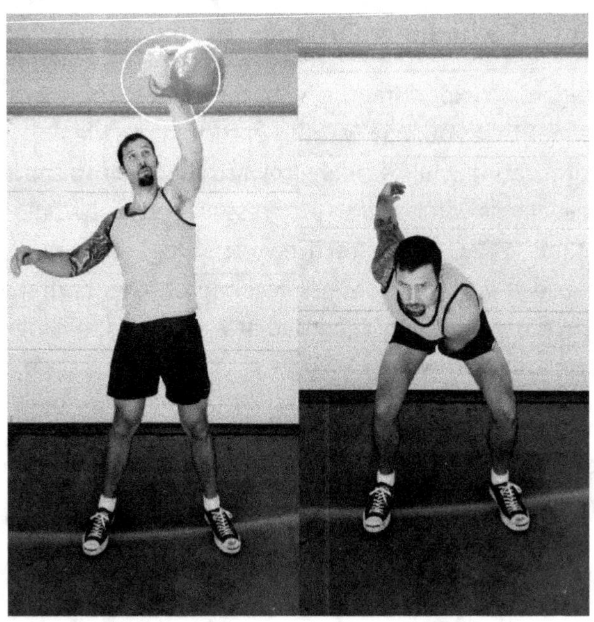

- When performing the concentric (upward) portion of the movement, raise **both** heels and come up on the toes while moving the weight upward. As you begin to work with heavier kettlebells in the territory of 36kg and beyond, you may find that keeping the heels planted while attempting to perform many repetitions can be quite strenuous on the lumbar and sacral areas of the low back. This one simple nuance can help with moving heavier weights for more repetitions while preventing strained discs and flare-ups in the sacroiliac (SI) joint.

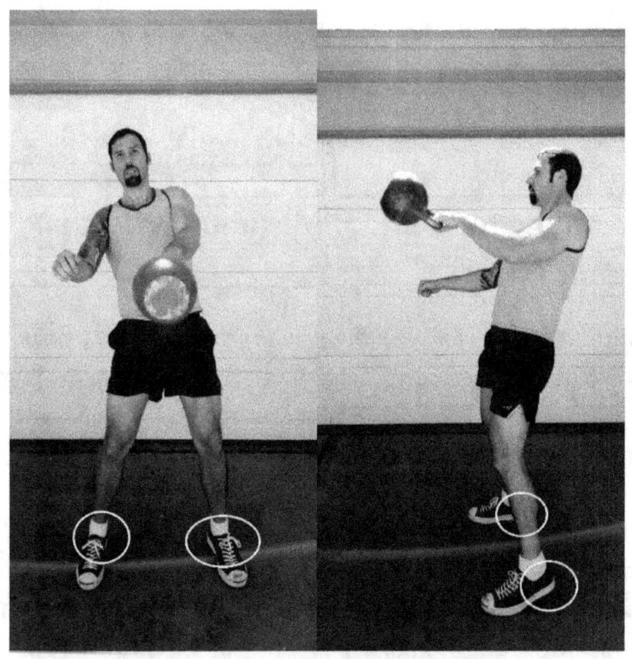

Just remember, in the context of training on your own there is really no such thing as "cheating." Don't be afraid to experiment or take liberties with certain aspects of an exercise even if it's not exactly "by the book" so long as you are not injuring yourself or doing something completely stupid. These ideas are **optional**, they do not have to be implemented unless you choose to do so.

By incorporating these methods with heavier kettlebells, you can harness the ability to move back down in weight and perform a 100 rep snatch test with perfect hardstyle technique using both a 24kg and 32kg kettlebell. If you intend on preparing for an instructor certification, it may be of use to experiment with these techniques using heavier weight and then perform the snatch test with your "test weight" to see where you stand. Always keep in mind that you will also need to perform the snatch within the requirements of the organization in the event that you wish to certify.

The Conjugate Method: Maximum Effort and Dynamic Effort

If you're at all familiar with the powerlifting world, the Westside Barbell club has produced more world records than any gym in the sport by using the "Conjugate Method" developed by Louie Simmons, widely considered as a genius in many respects when it comes to strength training and athletic performance. Although it isn't totally necessary to complete the 100-rep snatch test by using all of the concepts within the conjugate method, understanding the use of a maximum effort day and a dynamic effort day are particularly useful for what will be presented in later sections.

Two of the key components regarding the method that will be outlined can be described by two laws of physics: **1. Speed = Distance/Time (Distance = Speed x Time)** and **2. Force = Mass x Acceleration**. As Simmons once said, "You can't move a heavy weight slow." By decreasing the time in which repetitions are performed, we can cover greater distance in a shorter period of time. Likewise, by increasing the force by which a heavy weight can be moved for more repetitions, muscular contraction and the coordination of the kinetic chain will improve so that more repetitions can be performed with a lighter weight. Over the years, I've heard several athletes mention that they simply used a 28kg kettlebell to prepare for a snatch test to become certified if a 24kg kettlebell was their test weight. While this has the right intention, it doesn't quite go far enough in regard to the force development needed to make a lighter kettlebell become less challenging in comparison.

Because of the ballistic nature of the snatch, we will take some liberties with the conjugate method and incorporate one day in which speed and maximum effort are combined while a second day will serve to improve distance and/or repetitions. We will refer to them as a **Force Day** and **Distance Day** respectively.

Resistance Variables, Measurability, and Acclimation

Before continuing, I must set the expectation in regard to a few key points:

- The examples that are used will be **limited to 3 to 4 sets** of snatching. Generally speaking, less than 3 sets of snatching is not enough practice while more than 4 sets is too much. I have found this to be the sweet spot over the years in regard to fatigue management as well as preventing hand tears.
- In regard to rest between sets, the examples **will not exceed 3 minutes of rest between each set and they will not be less than 1 minute and 30 seconds**. More than 3 minutes between sets is not challenging enough while less than 1 minute and 30 seconds is too aggressive. When time between sets is too aggressive, it may need to be increased back to 3 minutes along with weight and/or repetitions needing to be increased at this point.
- In regard to repetitions, **Distance Days generally fall within the 15-25 rep range (per arm) while Force Days**

generally fall within the 5-12 rep range (per arm). Once 25 repetitions (50 total) have been met on Distance Days and 12 repetitions (24 total) have been met on Force Days for every set indicated, it may be time to consider increasing the weight and reverting back to the original starting point. Keep in mind that this may vary depending on when a plateau is reached.

- **All sets are limited to one hand switch without putting the kettlebell down.** The reason that multiple hand switches are not recommended is because it will completely throw off the programming efforts and make the entire process less measurable. As soon as multiple hand switches are introduced, the ability to quantify will deviate, and linear progression is of critical importance. By only performing one hand switch per set, it ensures that the strength and endurance of each hand and arm is developed evenly and efficiently. If you are having to switch multiple times or setting the bell down during a set, **the resistance variables are too challenging**. Make adjustments in order to decrease the resistance so that all sets and reps can be completed.
- When increasing repetitions on each set, **always increase the repetitions on both arms, never just one and not the other.** Similar to limiting each set to one hand switch, it makes little sense to do more repetitions on one arm than the other during a set as each arm should be developed evenly.
- When decreasing rest times between each set, **always strive to decrease each rest time by the same amount of seconds**. All rest times should be distributed as

evenly as possible. Generally speaking, **rest times should only be decreased by 5-10 seconds at a time.**

- During rest periods, **you can either remain standing or sit.** It is completely up to the athlete in regard to how they wish to utilize rest between sets as long as the next set begins exactly when the rest period ends.

The Rep-Goal Method

The Rep-Goal method is a very simple method in regard to progressive overload, which is implemented by determining what sets, reps, and weight you are comfortable with at the very beginning of your snatching journey and gradually adding one repetition to each set while keeping the rest in-between sets at a constant. The number of weight, sets, reps, and time that an athlete wants to start at can vary from one person to the next and is based upon how the individual feels. It is highly recommended to start at a threshold that can be performed **comfortably** so that the starting point can be accurately measured over time.

Let's say that for your Distance Day, you want to start with a 24kg kettlebell and perform 4 sets of 15 on each arm (20) total with 3 minutes rest between each set. It would look as follows:

Week	# Sets	# Reps	Rest Time	Weight
1	4	15 + 15 / 15 + 15 / 15 + 15 / 15 + 15	3:00	24kg

Once this can be completed **convincingly,** then it's simply a matter of adding a repetitions to sets over time:

Week	# Sets	# Reps	Rest Time	Weight
1	4	15 + 15 / ~~15 + 15~~ / 15 + 15 / 15 + 15	3:00	24kg
2	4	15 + 15 / 16 + 16 / 15 + 15 / 15 + 15	3:00	24kg

Eventually, you should come to a point where you have achieved the following as weeks have gone by:

Week	# Sets	# Reps	Rest Time	Weight
1	4	15 + 15 / ~~15 + 15~~ / 15 + 15 / 15 + 15	3:00	24kg
2	4	~~15 + 15~~ / 16 + 16 / 15 + 15 / 15 + 15	3:00	24kg
3	4	16 + 16 / 16 + 16 / ~~15 + 15~~ / 15 + 15	3:00	24kg
4	4	16 + 16 / 16 + 16 / 16 + 16 / ~~15 + 15~~	3:00	24kg
5	4	16 + 16 / 16 + 16 / 16 + 16 / 16 + 16	3:00	24kg

This example illustrates an improvement of **8 overall repetitions over 5 weeks**. Is it likely that everything will go according to plan over 5 weeks however? **Probably not.** You may have to repeat certain weeks until you proceed with adding two more repetitions to remaining sets. **It's all about acclimation.** In regard to how fast you choose to progress is completely up to you, but eventually you will find a sticking point where things become very challenging or you reach a plateau. It is up to you to determine what course of action you will take in order to break the barrier. This outline can be followed indefinitely until it becomes too challenging. In this illustration for example, once 25 repetitions per arm has been met on each set, it may be time to consider moving to a heavier weight and starting over again.

The Rest Interval Method

Unlike the Rep-Goal Method where repetitions are increased over time while rest times remain constant, the Rest Interval Method differs in that it involves decreasing the rest time in-between each set while keeping the weight constant.

Let's say that for your Force Day, you want to start with a 36kg kettlebell and perform 4 sets of 6 on each arm (12) total with 3 minutes rest between each set. It would look as follows:

Week	# Sets	# Reps	Rest Time	Weight
1	4	6 + 6 / 6 + 6 / 6 + 6 / 6 + 6	3:00	36kg

Once this can be completed **convincingly**, then it's simply a matter of decreasing the rest periods over time:

Week	# Sets	# Reps	Rest Time	Weight
1	4	6 + 6 / 6 + 6 / 6 + 6 / 6 + 6	~~3:00~~	36kg
2	4	6 + 6 / 6 + 6 / 6 + 6 / 6 + 6	2:55	36kg

Although a 5 second decrease to the rest period may not seem like much, you must consider that 4 sets are being performed. Therefore, it is an overall **15 second decrease** in regard to the work performed. Eventually, you should come to a point where you have achieved the following as weeks have gone by:

Week	# Sets	# Reps	Rest Time	Weight
1	4	6 + 6 / 6 + 6 / 6 + 6 / 6 + 6	~~3:00~~	36kg
2	4	6 + 6 / 6 + 6 / 6 + 6 / 6 + 6	~~2:55~~	36kg
3	4	6 + 6 / 6 + 6 / 6 + 6 / 6 + 6	~~2:50~~	36kg
4	4	6 + 6 / 6 + 6 / 6 + 6 / 6 + 6	~~2:45~~	36kg
5	4	6 + 6 / 6 + 6 / 6 + 6 / 6 + 6	2:40	36kg

This example illustrates an improvement of performing the overall workload in **1 minute less time**. Is it likely that everything will go according to plan over 5 weeks however? **Probably not.** You may have to repeat certain weeks until you proceed with decreasing the rest time. Again, **it's all about acclimation**. In regard to how fast you choose to progress is completely up to you, but eventually you will find a sticking point where things become very challenging or you reach a plateau. You have to keep working at the threshold that is challenging until it is no longer a challenge and you choose to move forward.

Putting It All Together

Now that we have reviewed the principles behind a force and distance day, the rep-goal method, and the rest interval method, let's review some scenarios in which each of them are incorporated. If you haven't figured it out already, **a timer will be your best friend.** Most cell phones have a timer function unless you choose to buy a cheap kitchen timer. Either way, it is of paramount importance that you time your sets. The chosen weights, sets, reps, and rest times are to be determined by the athlete at his or her own discretion. A general rule is that the "force weight" should be 12-16kg heavier than the "distance weight" to ensure that proper force development will carry over to the lighter weight over time.

In regard to how often you choose to snatch, it is recommend to do so twice a week with one day being a distance day and the other being a force day, at least at the beginning. It does not matter if you choose to work on force or distance first during the week. As time goes on and the resistance variables become more challenging, you may choose to only snatch once per week and alternate between Distance and Force every other week. Nevertheless, if progress stalls or even begins to regress, it is up to the athlete to determine if more or less training frequency is needed.

One important note: **Always perform warm-up sets prior to the first working set.** There shouldn't necessarily be any sort of rhyme or reason to warming up as long as it mentally and physically prepares you for engaging in the first working set as much as possible. This can even include doing 3-5 reps on each arm of a heavier weight than what will be used for the working sets and then coming back down in weight. By warming up to a heavier weight than the working sets and then coming back down, you may find that it wakes the body up much more efficiently in order to begin the first working set.

Scenario A – Rep-Goal Distance Day and Rep-Goal Force Day

In this scenario, we will presume that the athlete is training the snatch twice per week. Because of this, he or she will perform 3 sets rather than 4 sets in comparison to previous examples to ensure recovery each week. We will also presume that 2 minutes of rest between sets on the force day is sufficient to complete every repetition of every set. I must emphasize that while the overall concepts should be understood, the sets, reps, and rest times are up to the individual to determine in order to continue to break through plateaus and make progress.

Week	Session	# Sets	# Reps	Rest Time	Weight
1	Distance	3	15 + 15 / 15 + 15 / 15 + 15	3:00	24kg
1	Force	3	6 + 6 / 6 + 6 / 6 + 6	2:00	36kg

Hypothetically, we will say that all variables remained the same during week 2 and no adjustments were made until week 3:

Week	Session	# Sets	# Reps	Rest Time	Weight
1	Distance	3	15 + 15 / 15 + 15 / 15 + 15	3:00	24kg
1	Force	3	6 + 6 / 6 + 6 / 6 + 6	2:00	36kg
2	Distance	3	15 + 15 / ~~15 + 15~~ / 15 + 15	3:00	24kg
2	Force	3	6 + 6 / ~~6 + 6~~ / 6 + 6	2:00	36kg
3	Distance	3	15 + 15 / **16 + 16** / 15 + 15	3:00	24kg
3	Force	3	6 + 6 / **7 + 7** / 6 + 6	2:00	36kg

If you've noticed from the few examples that I've illustrated so far, the first set of increases when using the rep-goal method is applied to the **second set and/or middle sets**. When using this method, you may find that the middle sets ends up going smoother than the first set and last sets, with the first set essentially providing a sort of warm-up for the remaining workload. With that said, it's completely up to the individual in concern to where they choose to make increases first. After approximately seven weeks of progress, the athlete has finally arrived at this point:

Week	Session	# Sets	# Reps	Rest Time	Weight
7	Distance	3	16 + 16 / 16 + 16 / 16 + 16	3:00	24kg
7	Force	3	7 + 7 / 7 + 7 / 7 + 7	2:00	36kg

As progress continues, the athlete may begin to notice that the force development from the force day and the stamina development from the distance day begin to complement one another and improve performance on each day.

Scenario B – Rest Interval Distance Day and Rest Interval Force Day

In this scenario, we will presume that the athlete is more advanced and is training the snatch once per week. Because of this, he or she will perform total work 4 sets as opposed to 3. We will also presume that the rep-goal method on force day is too aggressive, opting for the rest interval method until further notice or until a plateau has been reached.

Week	Session	# Sets	# Reps	Rest Time	Weight
1	Distance	4	20 + 20 / 20 + 20 / 20 + 20 / 20 + 20	3:00	32kg
2	Force	4	8 + 8 / 8 + 8 / 8 + 8 / 8 + 8	3:00	48kg

As indicated, rather than both weeks being indicated as being Week 1, we have a Week 1 and Week 2 since the snatch is only being trained once per week. The kettlebells being used are significantly heavier as well. After some time has gone by, there have only been adjustments made during weeks 7 and 8:

Week	Session	# Sets	# Reps	Rest Time	Weight
5	Distance	4	20 + 20 / 20 + 20 / 20 + 20 / 20 + 20	3:00	32kg
6	Force	4	8 + 8 / 8 + 8 / 8 + 8 / 8 + 8	3:00	48kg
7	Distance	4	20 + 20 / 20 + 20 / 20 + 20 / 20 + 20	2:50	32kg
8	Force	4	8 + 8 / 8 + 8 / 8 + 8 / 8 + 8	2:55	48kg

You will notice that the adjustments to the time made to the force day is **less than** the adjustment made to the distance day, which is perfectly fine. As long as some sort of progress is being made to each session over time, they can be at variance with one another which will happen quite often. In a perfect world each day will progress at the same rate, but they almost never will unless you are in the beginning stages of programming the snatch. In fact, the athlete may run into a situation where one day out paces the other and they are able to start the rest time back over and increase repetitions on one day while still decreasing rest times on the other:

Week	Session	# Sets	# Reps	Rest Time	Weight
33	Distance	4	20 + 20 / 20 + 20 / 20 + 20 / 20 + 20	~~2:30~~	32kg
34	Force	4	~~8 + 8 / 8 + 8 / 8 + 8 / 8 + 8~~	~~2:00~~	48kg
35	Distance	4	20 + 20 / 20 + 20 / 20 + 20 / 20 + 20	2:25	32kg
36	Force	4	12 + 12 / 12 + 12 / 12 + 12 / 12 + 12	3:00	48kg

As indicated, the distance day is still continuing down the path of decreasing rest times while the athlete has chosen to increase the rest time back to the original 3 minutes and increase repetitions on force day, starting the process over again. As you become more advanced, you will find that it will be much more challenging to make increases and that you may have to start the process over sooner and/or more often.

Scenario C – Rep-Goal Distance Day and Rest Interval Force Day

In this scenario, the athlete has decided that increasing the repetitions during the distance day while keeping the rest constant will help to increase lung capacity over time. Additionally, the weight being used during the force day is a bit challenging to try to increase repetitions, therefore a decision has been made to decrease rest intervals while keeping the repetitions constant. The snatch will be trained twice per week. There are 3 sets during the distance day while there are 4 sets during the force day.

Week	Session	# Sets	# Reps	Rest Time	Weight
1	Distance	3	20 + 20 / 20 + 20 / 20 + 20	3:00	24kg
1	Force	4	7 + 7 / 7 + 7 / 7 + 7 / 7 + 7	2:00	40kg

In this example, you will notice that there is a 16kg difference in weight and we are working with sets of 7 during the force day. The sizes of kettlebells that you have available will play a big part in determining the overall setup. Personally, I have always worked with kettlebells that are at least 8kg apart in weight, so naturally the distance day and force day will typically involve a 16kg difference. As long as endurance is being trained on one day while force and explosiveness is being trained on the other, there will be progress as long as solid technique is being maintained and incremental improvements are recorded over time.

After 8 weeks, we will hypothesize that the athlete has made progress but has started running into problems:

Week	Session	# Sets	# Reps	Rest Time	Weight
7	Distance	3	23 + 23 / 23 + 23 / ~~22 + 22~~	3:00	24kg
7	Force	4	7 + 7 / 7 + 7 / 7 + 7 / 7 + 7	~~1:45~~	40kg
8	Distance	3	23 + 23 / 23 + 23 / 23 + 21 fail	3:00	24kg
8	Force	4	7 + 7 / 7 + 7 / 7 + 7 / 4 + 4 fail	1:35	40kg
9	Distance	3	23 + 23 / 23 + 23 / 22 + 22	3:00	24kg
9	Force	4	7 + 7 / 7 + 7 / 7 + 7 / 7 + 7	1:40	40kg

As indicated, when an increase of two reps were attempted on the distance day and a 10 second decrease was attempted on the force day, the athlete failed to meet goal on the last set. It is inevitable that this will happen from time to time if the athlete did not spend enough time acclimating to the previous numbers or if the increases made were a bit too much. Going into Week 9, the adjustment has been made to go back to the variables indicated for week 7 for distance day while decreasing the rest between sets by 5 seconds instead of 10 seconds on force day.

Continuing with this illustration, we will use a "perfect world" example where the end goals have been met at the same time after 30 weeks:

Week	Session	# Sets	# Reps	Rest Time	Weight
30	Distance	3	~~25 + 25 / 25 + 25 / 25 + 25~~	3:00	~~24kg~~
30	Force	4	~~7 + 7 / 7 + 7 / 7 + 7 / 7 + 7~~	~~1:30~~	~~40kg~~
1	Distance	3	15 + 15 / 15 + 15 / 15 + 15	3:00	32kg
1	Force	4	5 + 5 / 5 + 5 / 5 + 5 / 5 + 5	3:00	44kg

As indicated, the athlete has met the 25 rep goal on each set and has decided to increase the weight to 32kg and start at 15 repetitions per arm during each set for distance day. In addition, the 1:30 goal has been met during the force day and the decision has been made to increase the rest time up to 3 minutes and decrease the repetitions to 5 per set, increasing the weight to 44kg.

When the 25 rep goal during distance day, 12 rep goal during force day, or the 1:30 timeframe has been met, it is up to the athlete to determine how they would like to establish the new resistance variables and start the cycle over. It's also important to understand that the new variables may not always work upon the first attempt and may need to be adjusted with some experimentation. Keep in mind that a plateau could be reached before the ultimate rep goals and rest interval timeframe is met, and trying to reach them without starting over could be an exercise in futility.

Scenario D – Rest Interval Distance Day and Rep-Goal Force Day

In this scenario, the athlete has decided that decreasing the rest between sets while keeping the repetitions constant during the distance day will help to overcome lactic acid buildup in the wrist and forearms. Additionally, the athlete has a strong endurance threshold and wants to improve strength development, opting for increasing repetitions during force day while keeping the rest time at a constant 3 minutes. 4 sets for distance day and 3 sets for force day have been indicated, training twice per week.

Week	Session	# Sets	# Reps	Rest Time	Weight
1	Distance	4	15 + 15 / 15 + 15 / 15 + 15 / 15 + 15	3:00	12kg
1	Force	3	5 + 5 / 5 + 5 / 5 + 5	3:00	24kg

With the weights indicated here, more than likely the athlete is a female who has reached the intermediate stage of snatch development. Even if the chosen kettlebells are a lighter weight, the general principles that have been illustrated in previous examples remain intact. The rate of progress and recovery may be different, but the ultimate goal is to make progress nonetheless. We will assume the following progress after a 10 week period:

Week	Session	# Sets	# Reps	Rest Time	Weight
9	Distance	4	15 + 15 / 15 + 15 / 15 + 15 / 15 + 15	~~2:45~~	12kg
9	Force	3	7 + 7 / 7 + ~~7~~ / 7 + 7	3:00	24kg
10	Distance	4	15 + 15 / 15 + 15 / 15 + 15 / 15 + 15 barely met	2:40	12kg
10	Force	3	7 + 7 / 8 + 8 / 7 + 7	3:00	24kg

As indicated for the distance day on Week 10, the athlete barely met the goal for the last set which can mean a few different things. Either their form started breaking down during the last few repetitions, or it took everything they had to complete the set. This puts the athlete in a precarious position. My recommendation is that if the form started to break down slightly, it would be advisable to simply stay at this threshold until the set is no longer a struggle. If it required an all-out effort to complete the set, it would be more appropriate to increase the rest times back to where this does not occur. Likewise, if it is the rep-goal method rather than the rest interval method being used then the same reasoning would apply by decreasing the repetitions back down.

Supplemental Exercises

There are a variety of supplemental exercises that can be used to compliment the snatch and possibly replace them on occasion. This could arise when inflammation begins to occur, if progressing to a new weight is too heavy, or if a hand tear prevents the athlete from snatching efficiently. They are not required to perform by any means, but you may reach a point where they could be helpful. A brief overview will be provided in regard to these supplemental exercises and the benefits of each of them.

Half Snatch

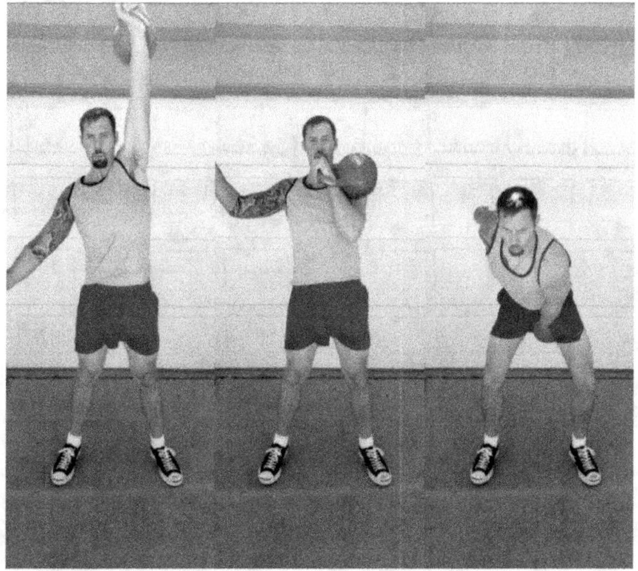

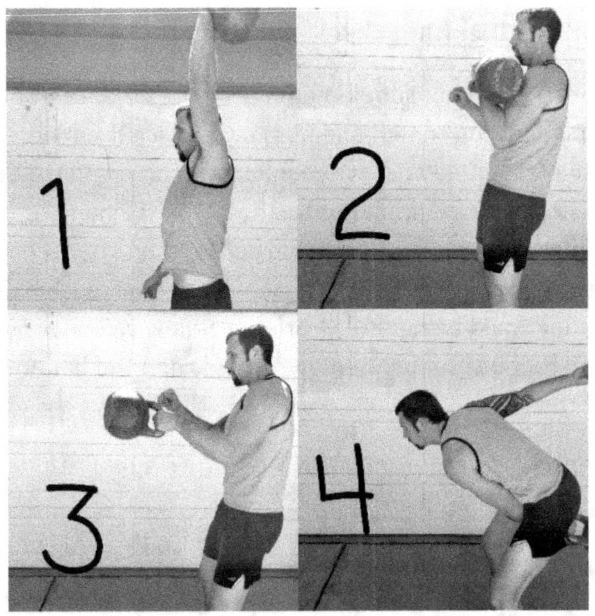

The half snatch deviates from the full snatch in one aspect: Rather than swinging the kettlebell from the overhead position all the way to the knees on the way down, the kettlebell is instead lowered into the finished clean or "rack" position, similar to the eccentric portion of an overhead press or jerk. Once the kettlebell has been lowered into the rack position, the kettlebell is then lowered to the knees and snatched all the way back up into the overhead position.

This is useful for two reasons:

- It prevents the hand from tearing as most hand tears occur on the way down.
- There are circumstances where the athlete will be strong enough to snatch a weight up, but will lose their

grip and the ability to control the kettlebell on the way
down.

The half snatch can be particularly useful and may serve as a substitution for a full snatch during force days, especially if the athlete is limited in regard to what kettlebell sizes that they have access to. For example, if a 44kg is not available and increasing from 40kg to 48kg is the only option, then performing the half snatch rather than the full snatch for explosive work can be extremely worthwhile. This can bridge the gap until the athlete gains the confidence to perform the full snatch. In fact, if the athlete **only wants to half snatch** once they reach a certain point, then it is perfectly acceptable so long as the force development is carrying over to distance days in addition to the snatch test using the "test weight." You would simply program the half snatch using the same methods that were outlined in the "Putting it All Together" section, although it is recommended to limit the half snatch to force day and continue to perform the full snatch during the distance day.

Burpees

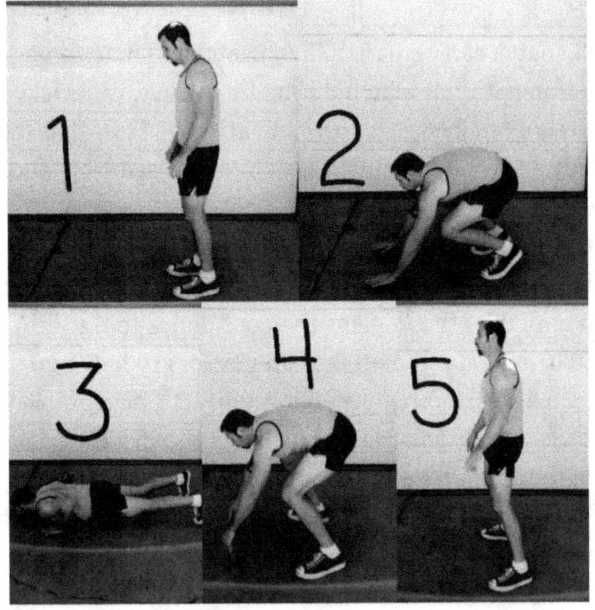

In addition to snatch programming, the ability to increase the number of burpees in addition to decreasing the amount of time that they are performed in can have tremendous carryover to the snatch. As long as the athlete does not have any debilitating injuries that prevents that from performing burpees, particularly in regard to the knees, they can be remarkably effective at increasing and maintaining muscular and cardiovascular endurance. There will be many situations in which a hand tear will prevent an athlete from being able to train the snatch, and burpees can be an excellent compensation if this occurs. Without elaborating too much, some worthwhile goals to consider are comprised of the following:

- 120 burpees in 10 minutes

- 160 burpees in 15 minutes
- 200 burpees in 20 minutes

This is also in regard to the variation of the burpee in which the legs come outside of the arms on the way up and the athlete simply rises to a standing position without jumping in the air at the end of each repetition. Burpee sets should be treated as "long distance" goals rather than "sprinting" goals so that they will carry over to the snatch effectively.

Sandbags

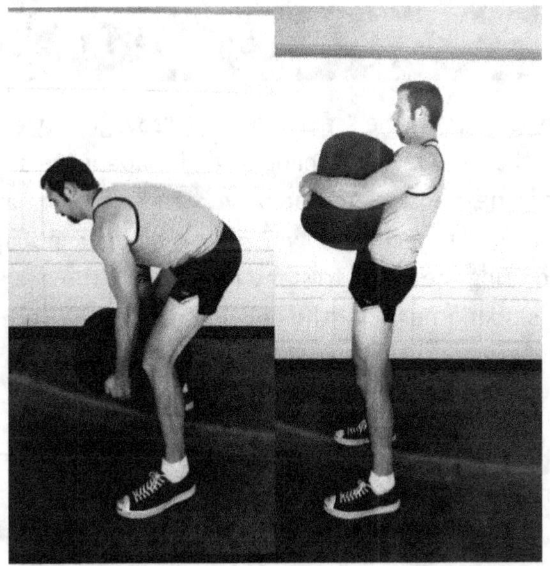

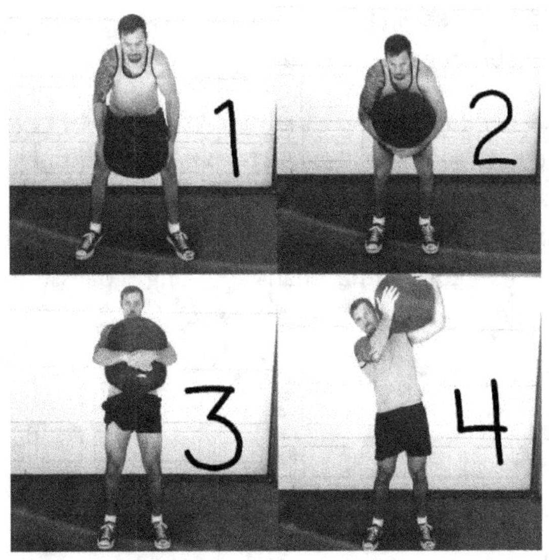

Sandbags, especially the "strongman" or "savage" style sandbags that are devoid of handles and shaped similar to atlas stones, are inexpensive and can be very corrective in nature. The simple act of reaching down and rowing the sandbag to the torso and using the knees to stand up with it in the bear hug position is phenomenal for the development of the core, glutes, and spinal erectors. There are different circuits that can be created with a sandbag, such as:

- Row-to-Bearhug: 6 sets of 6 with 150lb. sandbag, 1 minute rest between sets
- Alternating Belly-to-Shoulders: 10 sets of 4 with 150lb. sandbag, every minute on the minute
- Alternating Over-the-Shoulders: 8 sets of 6 with 150lb. sandbag, 2 minute rest between sets

The setups and possibilities are endless, and even if the sandbag is too light or too heavy you can always add or reduce the amount of sand that is stored within it. Sandbag circuits also share the same characteristic as burpees in the sense that they can be used as a compensation in the event that hand tears temporarily prevent the athlete from being able to snatch. It is also worth noting that if the athlete becomes more proficient with sandbag work, the spinal erectors and glutes will become much more coordinated so that SI joint inflammation and herniated discs are far less likely to occur.

Two Handed Swings

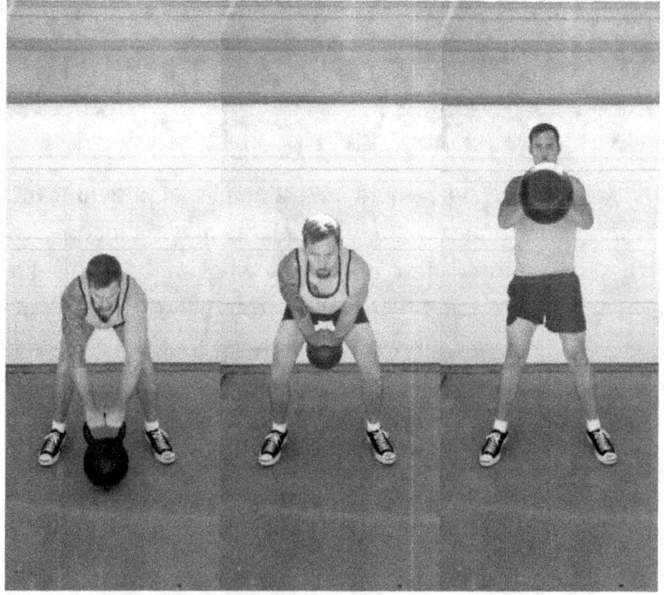

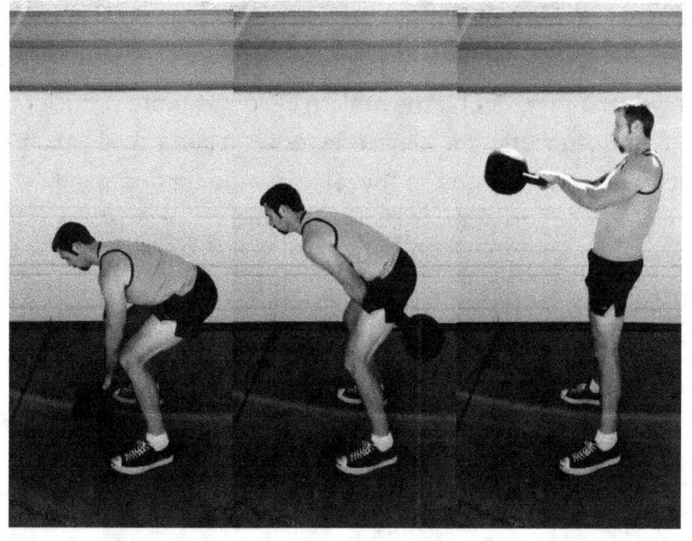

Heavy two handed swings with a kettlebell that is significantly larger than your typical snatching weights may be incorporated as an assistance movement during the week and can be a life saver in the event that inflammation from overuse occurs in the shoulders, wrists, and elbows. In the event that the athlete has a heavy bell such as a 48kg, 56kg, or 68kg, the snatch can be temporarily substituted with two handed swings until the inflammation goes away and snatch programming can resume as normal. It must also be noted that **one-handed swings are not recommended for this purpose.** The reason for this is because swinging with a single arm may contribute to worsening the inflammation whereas swinging with two hands will take pressure away from the problem areas and distribute the resistance evenly across the body.

A simple circuit such as 10 sets of 10 swings with 1-2 minutes of rest between each set can be a great starting point for two handed swings. Because of it's emphasis on building explosiveness in the glutes and quads, you may find that the snatch will be stronger when returning to it because of the increased leg drive that two handed swings will provide.

Single Leg Deadlift

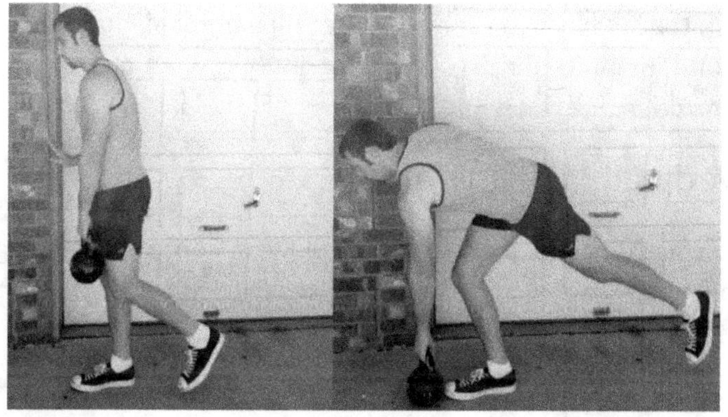

The glutes are a muscle group that can become quite dormant, especially if one's lifestyle outside of the training window is mostly sedentary. This is commonplace among individuals whose occupation involves sitting in a chair for the vast majority of their working hours. Single leg deadlifts with constant tension on the glute for high repetitions can be excellent for "waking up" the glutes and getting them to function properly, and they can be done nearly anywhere.

2-3 sets of 30-40 repetitions on each leg with a 20-24kg kettlebell will be more than sufficient for this purpose. The working arm should be the opposite arm of the working leg rather than using the arm and leg on the same side because it will put more tension on the glute by performing the movement this way. There should be a slight bend in the knee and the kettlebell should land in front of the toe on the way down. No pausing or locking out should occur at any point during the repetitions so that maximum stimulation can be channeled to the glute. If necessary, the non-working hand can hold onto a chair or the edge of a table to maintain balance while concentrating on the glute as much as possible.

Once the set has been complete, set the kettlebell down, walk around for a few minutes, and then do the same thing on the other side.

Overhead Mobility

There are many mobility exercises that can improve snatching proficiency, and two of these exercises in particular can help to address many problems.

Armbar

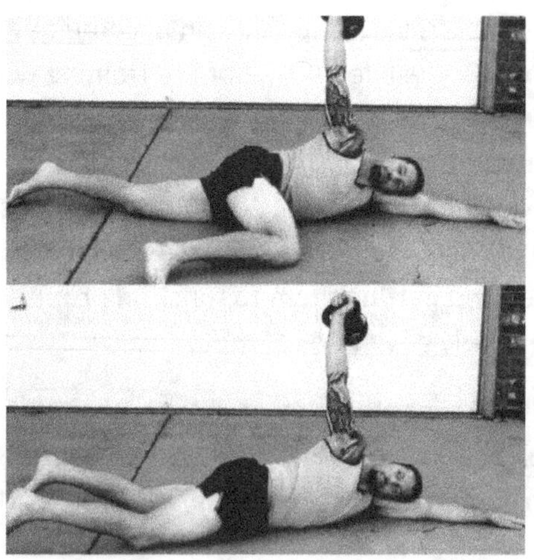

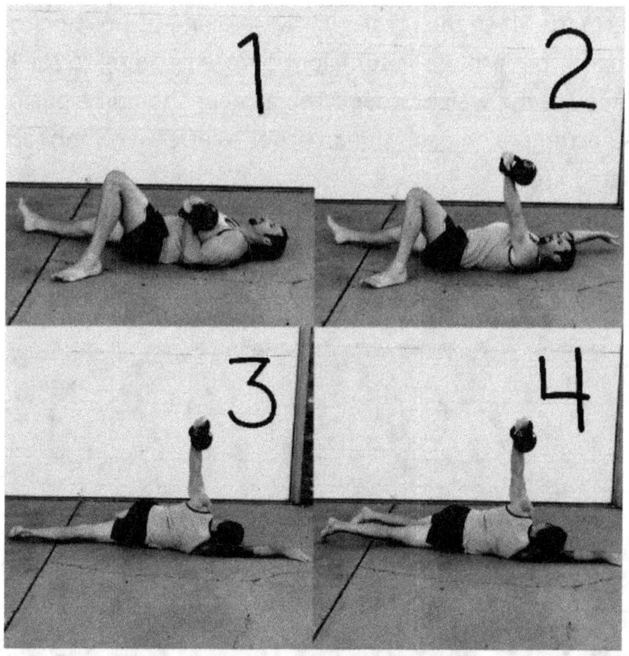

The armbar is typically performed with a weight light enough that it can be performed appropriately but heavy enough so that the body can be mobilized affectively. This can generally be around 12kg-16kg for men and 4-8kg for women, although the weight can be increased depending on strength and experience level. It is superb for improving thoracic mobility in the mid-back and increasing range of motion in the lumbar and sacral regions of the low back, diminishing the possibility of SI joint inflammation, herniated discs, neck injuries, or a winging scapula (jammed shoulder blade) from occurring.

In regard to improving overhead mobility for the snatch, it is recommended to "peel the lat" open on the non-working arm during the final step, relaxing the entire body on this area and striving to create more space in the teres minor region that connects the lat to the rotator cuff. Holding this position for 20-30 seconds per armbar is sufficient before deciding to roll back over and set the weight down. The armbar should be performed for 2-3 attempts on each side in order to effectively mobilize restricted areas.

Shoulder Dislocates

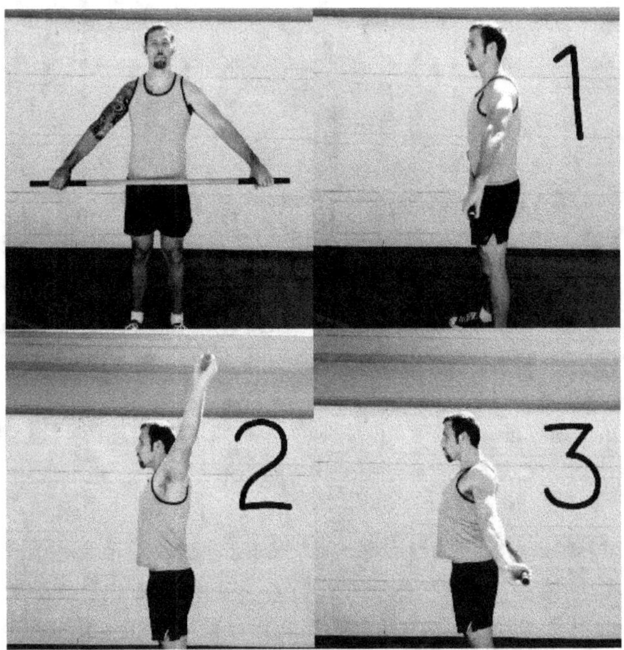

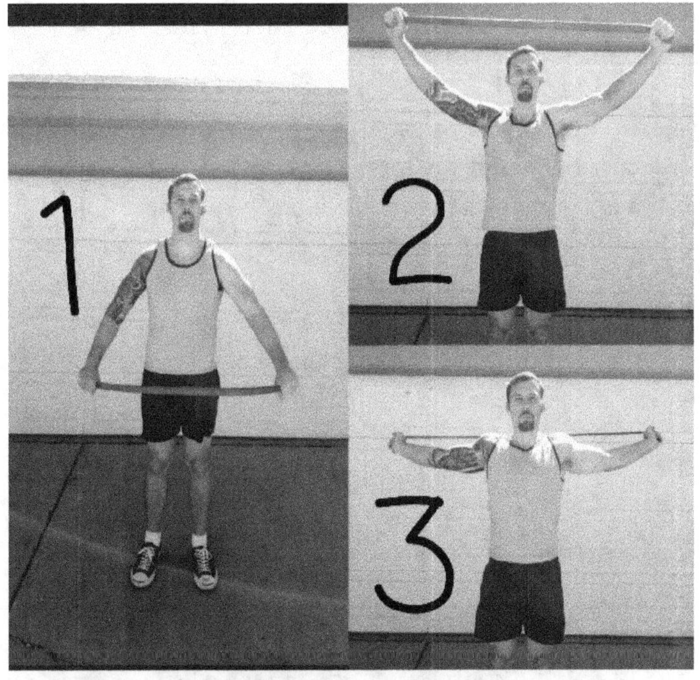

Shoulder dislocates, either with a mobility stick or a resistance band, can be a great way to work through restrictions in the pec minor, front deltoid, and scapular regions. These areas can become chronically tight from sitting in a chair or looking at a cell phone for many hours.

If you have a long wingspan, make sure that you are using a stick or a resistance band that can accommodate this so that you can start as wide as you need to in order to perform the movement effectively. The goal is to gradually bring your arms closer together over time. 5 sets of 10 repetitions can be an effective warm-up before a training session.

(Dis)honorable Mention: Double Snatch/Double Half Snatch

I will keep it short and simple by saying that **double snatching is only recommended if you intend on competing in Girevoy Sport.** It is a great exercise for developing and improving overhead fixation for the long cycle clean and jerk. However, double snatch variations can place a great deal of pressure on the knees and the low back. Unless the athlete intends on competing in sport, then the supplemental exercises previously mentioned are much safer alternatives for improving the one arm snatch.

Hand and Wrist Care

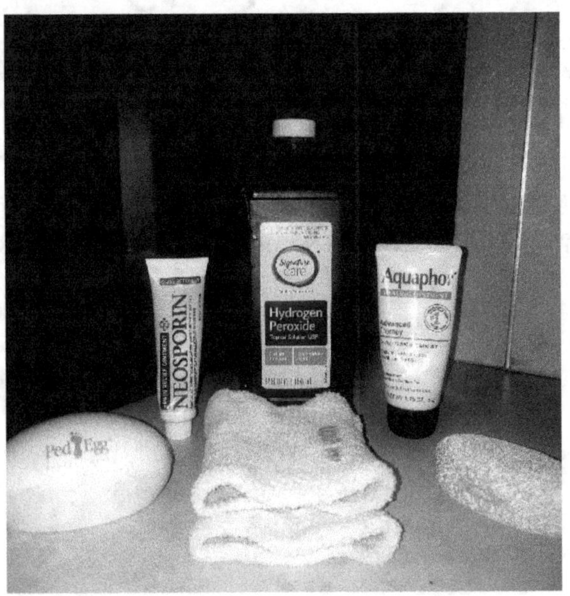

The snatch is notorious for building and tearing hand calluses which is why proper hand care is so critical. Although it is ideal to stop the set when you feel a blister or a tear begin to develop, it will happen on occasion. It should also be stated that **you should not shave too deeply or remove calluses altogether.** Although they are subject to tearing, calluses are extremely useful for preventing friction buildup while snatching a kettlebell. And no, wearing a pair of gloves is **not** an adequate substitute for gripping the handle of a kettlebell with bare hands. Any experienced kettlebell athlete will confirm this. The following products are highly recommended to have at your disposal:

- **PedEgg callus remover** – Although it is primarily used for feet, it can be used just as effectively for hand calluses. Over the years, I have found this to be the most reliable and longest lasting tool in regard to hand maintenance.
- **Pumice Stone** – Although not quite as efficient as a PedEgg, a pumice stone can sometimes shave off areas that are harder to reach with a PedEgg. Be careful not to create too much friction while using a pumice stone or you will create another blister around the area of concern.
- **Aquaphor** – This is an excellent moisturizer and is widely recommended for aftercare to prevent infection when a tattooed area of the body is still an open wound. After a hard snatching session, a layer of Aquaphor lathered onto the hands can help to soften up rough areas, especially if applied before going to sleep at night.

- **Hydrogen Peroxide/Neosporin/Bacitracin** – An antiseptic along with a pain relieving ointment should always be at your side when snatching regularly. In the event that a hand tear should occur, it is highly recommend to begin the healing process as soon as possible. Hydrogen peroxide is sufficient, but if you choose to use rubbing alcohol instead then I won't say that I didn't warn you.
- **Sweat Bands** – Sweat bands for the forearms can be a great thing to have when snatching frequently. As perspiration increases, the kettlebell will begin to rub against the forearms and cause sweat bumps to develop. This can become a distraction while attempting to improve the snatch, and wearing a pair of sweat bands will prevent this from occurring.

Conclusion - Frequency, Adjustments, and Recovery

While there is a general philosophy with specific guidelines to follow, it must be understood that there is going to be a great deal of nuance while working within the system. There are literally hundreds of scenarios that could be illustrated aside from what has been provided, and it is up to the athlete to uncover what that nuance happens to be on any given day, at any given moment, and make adjustments if needed, as needed. The primary focus is simply this: **Make small increases over time, keep record of them, know when to start over when a plateau has been reached, and stay injury free.** There is no magic number of sets, reps, rest times, or number of training days that can be followed as these resistance variables will evolve as the athlete continues to evolve. It is also useful to incorporate a week off or de-load weeks where the weight is reduced on occasion if the the nervous system needs a break or if active recovery is needed. This can also be a great opportunity to seek massage therapy or myofascial release using a foam roller.

After a substantial number of increases have been made, try testing your 100 rep snatch test in under 5 minutes with your snatch "test weight" **every 3 to 4 months and/or 12 to 16 weeks**. This will typically be within the range of 24kg - 28kg for men and 12kg - 16kg for women if you choose to base your desired snatch results upon the requirements of a certifying organization. You may be pleasantly surprised to find that your snatch has vastly improved, even if you can't meet the goal just yet. Eventually, you will reach a point where you can complete the test as if it were second nature.

Always remember that no matter how sound a training philosophy happens to be, **nothing works unless you do.** It will always require determination, will power, and the ability to think critically regardless of what system you choose to follow.

Happy Snatching!